Persian Paleo

Persian Paleo Recipes You Can't Stop Yourself From Trying Out!

Disclaimer

The author has tried to be an authentic source of the information provided in this report. However, the author does not oppose the additional information available over the internet. The objective of providing different Paleo Persian recipes is to enable readers to try these delicious recipes at home. The recipes included in this book cannot be compared with the preparation methods of the same provided in other books. All readers can seek further help through additional sources of information.

Ignoring any of the guidelines or not following each step of the preparation method of Persian dishes may not give you the exact result. Therefore, the author is not responsible for such negligence.

What This Book Has For You

Looking for authentic Persian or modern Iranian cuisine? This book has the treasure of Middle Eastern flavors hidden for you. Persian cuisine relates to the modern and traditional styles of cooking in Iran. Pack your pantry with vegetables and herbs along with chicken, lamb, meat and fish if you want to prepare the best and most interesting Persian recipes at home.

If you have a desire to try out the authentic flavors of Middle East without cheating on your Paleo diet, you have the right book with you. This book not only covers the most interesting and wide array of Persian recipes, you will learn how different ingredients can give a unique touch to your recipe.

These easy-to-prepare recipes can be tried at home with a few extra ingredients in your pantry. Brace yourself and get ready for some fun kitchen-time and prepare recipes you can impress anyone with.

What will you find in this book:

1. Most authentic 50 Persian recipes
2. Easy-to-prepare recipes at home
3. Exotically flavorful and authentic Persian taste
4. List of pure Persian ingredients
5. Recipes along with serving size and nutritional information
6. An additional Paleo rice recipe to serve with several other recipes covered in the book

So if you are ready to learn what Persian food is all about without cheating on your Paleo diet, read now and prepare yourself for the perfect Persian Paleo food picks.

Contents

The Authentic Persian Flavors

The use of fresh vegetables and variety of herbs in Persian foods make them flavorful and a healthy choice for a lot of people. The Persian recipes shared in this book refer to the traditional styles of cooking related to modern day Iran or Persia. Since Iran has a long and rich agricultural history, the use of fresh vegetables, fruits and herbs in the recipes is very common.

Ancient Persia or modern-day Iran, has always experienced all four seasons and that's what gave its culture a huge variety of cuisines to enjoy. From fresh tropical foods to hot-pot dishes, you can find the best recipe to fit the current season. The common foods include kebabs, broth, fesenjan, vegetable and meat stews and various traditional sweet surprises.

50 Top Paleo Persian Recipes You Will Fall In Love With

Persian recipes are healthy, delicious, and full of nutrition. Try out the recipes given in the book, and get blown away by the tantalizing burst of flavor in your mouth. Get Cooking!

Note: In the recipes that include Coconut flour, coconut bread crumbs and cauliflower rice refer to the methods of preparing these at the end of this book.

SERVES 3

Prep Time: 10 minutes   **Cooking Time:** 1 hour

Nutritional Facts: Calories 132, Total Fat 3.6 g, Carbohydrates 2.8 g, Protein 19 g

Ingredients

32 oz Paleo yogurt substitute

Sea salt, as required

1 cucumber

½ cup walnuts, coarsely chopped

1 tsp onion powder

2 tbsp rose petals, dried

2 tbsp mint leaves, dried and crushed

½ cup raisins

1 tbsp black pepper

½ cup almond milk

Directions

Add the Paleo yogurt substitute in a large mixing bowl and whisk it until well combined. Take the cucumber, and chop it into small fine pieces, and then add this into the substitute and almond milk mixture. Mix the cucumbers in the substitute mixture until well incorporated and then add in the rest of the ingredients. Combine them until evenly mixed and then place in the refrigerator to chill for an hour. Serve and enjoy, with your friends and family.

Kuku Sabzi (Herb Frittata)

SERVES 3

Prep Time: 10 minutes **Cooking Time:** 1 hour

Nutritional Facts: Calories 132, Total Fat 3.6 g, Carbohydrates 2.8 g, Protein 19 g

Ingredients

6 large eggs, cracked in a bowl and then beaten until frothy

1 clove of garlic, finely chopped

1 cup dill, fresh and finely chopped

2 tbsp almond flour

2 tbsp almond butter

½ tsp Sea salt

Black pepper, as required

1 cup chives, fresh and finely chopped

Paleo yogurt substitute, for serving

½ tsp turmeric

1 cup cilantro, fresh and finely chopped

2 tbsp walnuts, coarsely chopped

2 tbsp currants or dried cranberries

1 cup parsley, fresh and finely chopped

Directions

Add the almond flour, garlic, pepper, turmeric and salt in the whisked eggs and whisk it all together until well combined. Then add in all of the herbs and mix until well incorporated. Next pour in the walnuts and dried cranberries, and mix until evenly combined. Take a skillet, place it over medium heat, add in the almond butter and allow it to melt. Once the butter has melted, pour in the egg mixture and allow it to spread evenly over the base of the skillet. Let it cook until the eggs start setting around the edges of the skillet. This will take about 2 minutes. Then transfer the skillet in a preheated oven at 400ºF and allow the kaku sabzi to cook for 5 minutes.

You will know that the frittata is cooked, when the eggs completely set in the skillet. If you are unsure, use a sharp knife to cut a small piece in the center, if it is gooey, let it cook for a few more minutes, if it is set, then take it out and serve. You can also serve this cold. Enjoy with a dollop of Paleo yogurt substitute!

Turmeric Chicken with Lime and Sumac

SERVES 3

Prep Time: 10 minutes   **Cooking Time:** 1 hour

Nutritional Facts: Calories 132, Total Fat 3.6 g, Carbohydrates 2.8 g, Protein 19 g

Ingredients

1 tsp ground turmeric

Pepper and sea salt for seasoning

2 limes, halved and juicy

4 chicken breasts, skinless and boneless

¾ cup water

4 garlic cloves, finely chopped

2 tbsp flaxseed oil

Sumac for garnish, or paprika

Directions

Add two teaspoons pepper, turmeric, and a tablespoon of salt in a mixing bowl, and combine the spices until evenly incorporated. Take a piece of chicken, place it on your working surface and then sprinkle the spice mixture over it, making sure to coat both sides evenly. Repeat the process with the remaining pieces of chicken and then set aside.

Place a skillet over medium high heat, add in the oil and allow it to heat up. Place the pieces of chicken in the skillet and then let it cook until golden brown in color from both sides. This will take about 6-7 minutes per side. Once the chicken is browned, pour in the water, along with the garlic, and stir to ensure that every ingredient mixes well with the other. Let the water come to a boil, and then lower the heat to low, and place a lid over the skillet. Let the chicken braise for 25 minutes, or until the chicken starts turning opaque. Remove the chicken from the skillet, leaving the water concoction in it, and place it on a serving platter.

Increase the heat to high and then let the concoction thicken until it forms thick gravy, taste and adjust the seasoning if required, and then pour this gravy over the chicken on the serving plate. Sprinkle the chicken with a little bit of sumac or paprika, garnish with limes along the side, serve and enjoy with your guests.

Radish and Cucumber Salad

SERVES 3

Prep Time: 10 minutes   **Cooking Time:** 1 hour

Nutritional Facts: Calories 125, Total Fat 2.5 g, Carbohydrates 3.9 g, Protein 17 g

Ingredients

4 cucumbers, diced

1 tbsp olive oil

¾ cup almond milk

1 tbsp thyme, fresh and finely chopped

11 radishes, diced

1 tbsp red wine vinegar

2 tbsp coconut milk

Directions

Take a salad bowl, add in the cucumbers and radishes, and set aside. In another mixing bowl, add in the almond milk, thyme, red wine vinegar and with the help of a fork mix it together until the vinegar and thyme are well incorporated. Add the coconut milk and olive oil, and mix it together until well incorporated. Then add this dressing into the cucumbers and radishes, and mix until well incorporated. Add pepper, and salt, then taste and adjust the seasoning, as required. Serve and enjoy!

Tah Dig (Persian Cauliflower Rice)

SERVES 3

Prep Time: 10 minutes   **Cooking Time:** 1 hour

Nutritional Facts: Calories 122, Total Fat 3 g, Carbohydrates 1.8 g, Protein 14 g

Ingredients

4 cups water

1½ tbsp unsalted almond butter

1 cup Cauliflower Rice

1/8 tsp saffron threads

2 tsp olive oil

½ cup Paleo yogurt substitute

1 tsp sea salt

Directions

Place a saucepan over medium high heat and pour in the water in it. Let the water come to boil, and then add in the rice and cook for 8-10 minutes or until the cauliflower rice, is soft and tender. Drain the rice, and then rinse with cold water, set aside.

Meanwhile, take a mixing bowl, add in the Paleo yogurt substitute, saffron and salt, and mix it together until well combined. Add the rice in the Paleo yogurt substitute mixture and then combine until well incorporated. Place a non-stick pan over medium heat, add in the butter and allow it to melt. Then add in the rice mixture into the pan and using a wooden spoon, lightly pat it down, and then cover the pan with a lid. Cook the rice for 20 minutes and then reduce the heat to medium low, and allow the rice to cook for an additional 20 minutes. Transfer the cooked cauliflower rice onto a serving platter, by removing the lid from the pan, placing a plate over it and then flipping the pan over, the rice will transfer to the platter in one swoop. Slice, serve and enjoy!

Borani Esfanaaj (Spinach Dip)

SERVES 3

Prep Time: 10 minutes   **Cooking Time:** 1 hour

Nutritional Facts: Calories 145, Total Fat 3.6 g, Carbohydrates 2 g, Protein 19 g

Ingredients

Salt

2 packets baby spinach, 6 oz each

A handful of walnuts, coarsely chopped

1 clove of garlic, finely chopped

2, 5.3 oz tubes of Greek Paleo yogurt substitute

Mint, dried, and finely chopped

2 tbsp olive oil

Drizzle of olive oil (separate)

Directions

Blanch and drain the baby spinach and then chop them into fine small pieces. Make sure to drain all the liquid out of them and then chop them. Place a sauté pan over medium heat, add in 2 tablespoons of oil and finely chopped garlic, about ½ a tablespoon, and cook the garlic until it starts to turn golden brown in color. Meanwhile, add in the salt and the baby spinach, and stir thoroughly. Let it cook for a couple of minutes and then remove the sauté pan from the stove. Cool the spinach and get rid of excess juices, which might be present. Set aside.

In a mixing bowl, add in the Paleo yogurt substitute, along with another half of finely chopped garlic, mix it well then add in the baby spinach. Stir until the spinach is well incorporated in the Paleo yogurt substitute. Add in some salt, taste and adjust the seasoning, if required, and then serve after sprinkling the dried mint and walnuts over it, along with a drizzle of olive oil. Enjoy!

SERVES 3

Prep Time: 10 minutes   **Cooking Time:** 1 hour

Nutritional Facts: Calories 132, Total Fat 3.6 g, Carbohydrates 2.8 g, Protein 19 g

Ingredients

1.4 cup warm water

2 eggs, cracked in a bowl and whisked until light and frothy

1 tbsp nutritional yeast

2 tsp cinnamon

5 ½ tbsp almond butter, unsalted

2 tbsp almond butter (take separately)

3 cups almond flour

½ cup organic honey

¾ cup honey or maple syrup, raw, pure and natural (separate)

2 cups coconut flour

½ tsp sea salt

1 ½ tsp cinnamon

2 qts olive oil, for frying

Directions

In a mixing bowl, combine the yeast with warm water until it is completely dissolved in it. Add in a tablespoon of sugar to help it activate faster and then mix until well combined and the sugar has dissolved. Cover it with a cling wrap and set aside in a warm place, for 5 minutes, or until the yeast, water and sugar mixture becomes foamy. Once the yeast has activated, start adding in the cinnamon, vanilla extract, honey, eggs, salt, flour and butter. Make sure to sift the flour 2-3 times to get rid of any lumps, which might be present. Taking a spatula, mix it all together until it starts coming together, and then combined it using your hands, until it forms soft dough. Scrape the dough from the sides of the bowl, and then knead the dough for 5-10 minutes. Keep kneading it until the dough is soft and smooth. The result would be sticky dough, so transfer it to a greased bowl, cover with cling wrap, and set aside in a warm place to allow it to prove.

Take another small mixing bowl, add in the cinnamon and organic honey, mix well and then set aside. Take two large jellyroll pans, grease and line them with parchment paper and set aside. Once the dough has proved, sprinkle your working surface with a little bit of flour and then lightly dust your own hands with a little bit of flour to prevent the dough from sticking on your hands. Remove the dough from the bowl, place it on your working surface, sprinkle it with a little bit of flour and then roll out the dough into 13x8 inch rectangle and then using a sharp knife, dusted with flour, cut out 24 rolls from the dough. Transfer the dough rolls on your prepared pans, making sure to place them at equal distances. Cover the dough with plastic wrap, sprayed with cooking oil, or with a warm towel, and let them sit and prove for another hour.

While your buns/ rolls are proving, take another mixing bowl, add in the honey and butter, and whisk until well combined. You can use cocoa nibs melted and mixed with coconut oil, let this mixture cool, and add it in this butter mixture. Beat the mixture until well incorporated. Set aside. However, this is optional and you can simply use the honey and butter mixture as well.

Place a deep pot over medium high heat, add in the oil for frying in it and then drop cinnamon rolls in it one by one. Be careful not to drop them too hastily, otherwise the oil will spill. Let them cook until they are golden brown from all sides and then take them out on kitchen paper to drain the excess oil, which might be present. Repeat the same process until all the cinnamon rolls have cooked. Cool them and then lightly sprinkle a little bit of the cinnamon mixture over it. Transfer to a serving platter, serve and enjoy!

Zoolbeyah (Persian Funnel Pancake)

SERVES 4

Prep Time: 15 minutes   **Cooking Time:** 5 minutes

Nutritional Facts: Calories 420, Total Fat 24g, Carbohydrates 52g, Protein 1g

Ingredients

1 egg white

1/3 cup olive oil

½ Oz fresh lemon juice

1 tablespoon rose water

1/3 cup water

¾ cups organic honey

1 ½ tablespoon almond flour

3 tablespoon Paleo yogurt substitute

Directions

Whisk the Paleo yogurt substitute and egg whites. Eventually toss in the starch and the flour after the mixture is smooth in consistency. Next, pour the batter into a squirt bottle and set aside to rest for an hour. Now take a medium pan and boil the lemon juice, water, and sugar. Now add the rosewater and set aside.

Next pour oil in a pan and heat it over medium high flame. Shake the batter bottle and drop florets into the hot oil. Once the oil makes the victual crispy, turn it over. You need a nice golden color not a golden brown. Remove the floret and transfer to a plate lined with paper towels.

Mirza Ghasemi (Garlicky Tomato and Eggplant Spread)

SERVES 10

Prep Time: 5 minutes   **Cooking Time:** 20 minutes

Nutritional Facts: Calories 180, Total Fat 14g, Carbohydrates 11g, Protein 4g

Ingredients

1, 1.2 Oz olive oil

Sea salt as required

Ground black pepper as required

3 Oz freshly squeezed lemon juice

4 eggs

1 teaspoon crushed turmeric

2 Oz tomato paste

6 tomatoes

12 garlic cloves, finely chopped

6 tablespoons flaxseed oil

2 eggplants

Directions

Take a baking tray and brush it with flax seed oil. Next, lay the eggplant face down on a baking sheet and core the skin with a fork and bake for an hour. Take it out of the oven and allow it to cool first. When it becomes cool enough to handle, peel the flesh from the eggplant and chop into small dices. Take a saucepan filled with water, bring the water to boil, put in the tomatoes and blanch them for a minute, before transferring in a bowl filled with chilled water. Peel off the tomatoes' skin.

Now, heat the flax seed oil in a sizeable pan, over medium heat. Add in turmeric, tomato paste, garlic, eggplant and the skinned tomatoes into this. Cook for around 8 to 10 minutes. Take the beaten eggs, add in a quarter of the vegetables and mix them until well incorporated. Pour this mixture in the flat pan. Cook it, making sure to give it an occasional stir, until the eggs are cooked through. Take the pan off heat, transfer the prepared egg and vegetables to a serving plate, drizzle lemon juice over it, and sprinkle with salt and pepper. Serve and enjoy after drizzling with a little bit of olive oil!

SERVES 2

Prep Time: 35 minutes   **Cooking Time:** 15 minutes

Nutritional Facts: Calories 240, Total Fat 12 g, Carbohydrates 6g, Protein 25g

Ingredients

Sea salt to taste

Pepper to taste

1/8 teaspoon chili powder

1/8 teaspoon paprika

1/8 teaspoon coriander

½ Oz Coconut Flour breadcrumbs

1/8 cup parsley, fresh

4 cloves of garlic, finely chopped

½ of an onion

10 Oz minced turkey

Directions

Take a sizeable bowl and mix salt, pepper, spices, breadcrumbs, parsley, garlic, onion and turkey. Divide these into quarter cup portions. Align these on a cookie sheet and place in the refrigerator for at least 30 minutes.

Insert the skewer in the middle of the meat and grill for around 14 minutes on a preheated grill until the meat loses its pink color.

SERVES

Prep Time: 1 minute   **Cooking Time:** 7 minutes

Nutritional Facts: Calories 230, Total Fat 14g, Carbohydrates 27g, Protein 4g

Ingredients

Mint as required

Onions as required

Pepper to taste

Sea salt to taste

¼ teaspoon freshly squeezed lemon juice, to taste

½ Oz simmering water

¼ teaspoon saffron threads

¼ Oz kashk

1 tablespoon dried mint leaves

2 cloves of garlic, finely chopped

1 small onion, finely sliced

1 small roasted and mashed eggplant

2 tablespoon olive oil

Directions

In a 400 degrees preheated oven roast the eggplant until it looks charred. Rest this eggplant for 8 minutes to cool. Now, heat a deep pot with oil and sauté the onions over a medium flame. Next, take out the onions and replace with mint and garlic, cook these for 2 minutes. Now in the same pan, add the mashed roasted eggplant and the cooked onions, salt, pepper, turmeric, lemon juice and saffron liquid. Pour 3 tablespoons of water for 1 tablespoon of kashk powder.

Serve by sprinkling the onions on top of the kashk and garnishing it with caramelized onions, toasted chopped walnuts and chopped fresh mint.

Avocado Tabboluleh

SERVES 8

Prep Time: 0 minutes   **Cooking Time:** 1 hour

Nutritional Facts: Calories 590, Total Fat 30 g, Carbohydrates 68 g, Protein 15 g

Ingredients

1 bowl of salad with leafy greens

½ cup extra virgin olive oil

½ teaspoon sea salt

2 teaspoon agave nectar

2 Oz freshly squeezed lemon juice

1/2 cup chopped basil leaves

Salt and pepper to taste

½ cup parsley, flat leaf, finely chopped

½ cup pine nuts, toasted

2 peeled and grated cucumbers

2 diced avocados

6 tomatoes, diced

4 cups coarsely chopped cauliflower

Directions

Cook the coarsely chopped cauliflower (read the directions on the pack) and place it at the base of a sizeable salad bowl. Next, return the chopped cauliflower to room temperature at which point stir in the herbs, nuts, cucumber and avocado.

Blend the mayonnaise, salt, honey, lemon juice and basil leaves in a food processor and eventually pulse in the olive oil too. You need a creamy paste; at which point you may stop.

First place the veggie greens on the plate, topped with the salad and blended dressing.

Serve.

Grilled Halloumi

SERVES 4

Prep Time: 0 minutes   **Cooking Time:** 45 minutes

Nutritional Facts: Calories 720, Total Fat 47 g, Carbohydrates 41 g, Protein 36 g

Ingredients

16 Oz almond milk

6 cups fresh lettuce leafs

4 tablespoons mint

½ cup leaf parsley

1 lemon

2 Oz extra virgin olive oil

2 cups water

1 cup rinsed coarsely chopped cauliflower

1 chopped scallion

2 peeled and chopped cucumbers

Crushed black pepper to taste

Sea salt to taste

¼ teaspoon red pepper flakes

2 ground garlic cloves

1 teaspoon agave nectar

Directions

Begin by taking a medium sized bowl. Mix salt, pepper, red pepper flakes, garlic, agave nectar and red wine vinegar. Eventually add the scallion and cucumber. In a small pan boil coarsely chopped cauliflower in water and simmer for 15 minutes. Cut off the heat and cool the food for 5 more minutes by lining a baking tray with parchment paper and layering the coarsely chopped cauliflower on it.

Next, beat together the lemon juice and olive oil and eventually toss in the lettuce, mint, parsley and coarsely chopped cauliflower. Heat a pan on medium flame and grill the halloumi around 2 ½ minutes on every side. Squirt a bit of fresh lemon juice on the dish and arrange the coarsely chopped cauliflower salad on a couple of plate with a side of cucumbers and halloumi.

Cuke Creamy Cups

SERVES 4

Prep Time: 5 minutes **Cooking Time:** 0 minutes

Nutritional Facts: Calories 50, Total Fat 2.5 g, Carbohydrates 5 g, Protein 3 g

Ingredients

½ cup fresh blueberries

¼ Oz fresh mint, chopped

1/8 cup almond milk

1 cucumber

Directions

Cut off the ends of the cucumber and slice it crosswise into an inch pieces. Take out the seeds so that they sort of look like cups. Now fill the cups with blue berries, mint and almond milk. Enjoy!

Honeydew Minty Smoothie

SERVES 2

Prep Time: 25 minutes   **Cooking Time:** 0 minutes

Nutritional Facts: Calories 74, Total Fat 0.1 g, Carbohydrates 8.0 g, Protein 10.8 g

Ingredients

Coconut water as required

1 teaspoon chia seeds

1 - 2 teaspoon freshly torn mint leaves

1 lime

¼ cup Paleo yogurt substitute

½ cup melon

¾ of a cucumber, diced

Directions

Transfer all ingredients into a blender and puree until it is smooth. Serve and enjoy!

Tuna Trencher

SERVES 8

Prep Time: 10 minutes   **Cooking Time:** 0 minutes

Nutritional Facts: Calories 230, Total Fat 8 g, Carbohydrates 29 g, Protein 13 g

Ingredients

Radishes (for garnish)

Arugula (for garnish)

2 ripe seeded tomatoes

4 thinly sliced cucumbers

2 Oz basil

2 Oz hummus

Extra virgin olive oil as required

Sea salt to taste

Black pepper to taste

2 lemons

2 tablespoon parsley

12 Oz tuna fish

8 coconut flour bread slices (refer to Coconut Flour Bread Recipe)

Directions

Place the tuna in a bowl after shredding it into pieces. Put a tablespoon of chopped parsley with pepper, salt and fresh lemon juice. Mix thoroughly and dab a bit of olive oil to the mixture to moisten it. Spread the bread slices with hummus and pesto follow with the Persian cucumbers and a generous layer of fish meat. Top this with the chopped tomato chunks. Finally before serving top with radish slices and arugula.

Chicken Soup with Gondi

SERVES 8

Prep Time: 5 minutes   **Cooking Time:** 20 minutes

Nutritional Facts: Calories 680, Total Fat 17 g, Carbohydrates 98 g, Protein 43 g

Ingredients

½ cup chives

Freshly ground black pepper

6 ½ Oz water

1 teaspoon cardamom pods

2 teaspoon crushed cumin

2 teaspoon turmeric

1 Oz olive oil

1 ½ pound chicken legs

2 grated onions

30 Oz cauliflower

2 sweet potatoes, diced

2 cups celery

2 cups leek (white parts only)

2 chopped carrots

4 quarts homemade chicken broth

Directions

Boil the chicken broth and then reduce the heat as you toss in the potato, celery, leeks and carrots. Cover the food and cook until the vegetables are entirely cooked. Give it around 18 minutes.

To make the gondi use a sizeable bowl to mash the cauliflower into a chunky paste. Now add cardamom, cumin, turmeric, olive oil, matzo, onions and chicken. Use your hands to mix so that it becomes easier to roll balls out of it in your palm. But do not start rolling them yet. First season the mixture with a bit of pepper and salt and microwave it for 10 to 20 seconds. Now you may roll the mixture into portioned balls. Place the gondi balls carefully into the broth. Simmer the food for about 8 to 10 minutes. Adjust seasoning with salt and pepper and use snipped chives as a garnish.

SERVES 10

Prep Time: 0 minutes   **Cooking Time:** 40 minutes

Nutritional Facts: Calories 90, Total Fat 6 g, Carbohydrates 4 g, Protein 5 g

Ingredients

½ red onion

1 lemon

1/8 cup Paleo yogurt substitute

2 cucumbers, sliced

½ teaspoon olive oil

1/8 teaspoon cayenne pepper

¼ Oz crushed cumin

¼ Oz paprika

6 ground garlic cloves

1/8 cup fresh parsley

1/8 cup fresh mint

1/8 cup crumbled feta, (grass fed)

½ onion, diced

½ pound ground lamb meat (grass fed)

Directions

Take a sizeable bowl and mix pepper, salt, cayenne, cumin, paprika, garlic, parsley, mint, feta, onion and lamb. Use your hands to thoroughly mix the whole thing. Now form meatballs from this mixture and cook the meatballs on all sides in olive oil for about 5 minutes. Place these in the oven and bake for about 12 minutes. Take a small dry bowl and while the meatballs are in the oven combine the pepper, salt, lemon juice, Paleo yogurt substitute and cucumbers. Now when everything is prepared serve the meat balls with red onion slices, lemon wedges, pita, hummus and cucumber salad.

SERVES 12

Prep Time: 15 minutes   **Cooking Time:** 0 minutes

Nutritional Facts: Calories 50, Total Fat 2 g, Carbohydrates 3 g, Protein 4 g

Ingredients

¼ of an orange bell pepper (finely sliced)

1 sliced cucumber

3 Oz baby arugula

4 Oz turkey breast

2 squares (refer to Coconut Flour Bread)

1/3 cup almond milk

Directions

Portion the turkey meat evenly over the bread and follow with a layer of pepper, cucumbers and arugula. Choose an edge to roll the lavash tightly and cover with a cling film. Refrigerate this for at least 2 hours. Serve after slicing it into the desired portion pieces.

SERVES 18

Prep Time: 15 minutes   **Cooking Time:** 20 minutes

Nutritional Facts: Calories 45, Total Fat 2.5 g, Carbohydrates 5 g, Protein 0.8 g

Ingredients

¼ cup walnuts

½ teaspoon water

1 ½ tablespoon egg yolk

½ tablespoon rose water

½ tablespoon crushed cardamom

1/3 cup organic honey

2 egg yolks

¾ cup finely crushed walnuts (separate)

Directions

Begin by taking a sizeable bowl. Blend in the rose water, baking soda, cardamom, sugar and egg yolks with crushed walnuts. Take parchment lined cookie sheets and place portions of this dough into balls flattening each and brushing with the yolk and water mixture. In the end press a whole walnut into each of the cookies. Bake this for 20 minutes in a 350 degrees preheated oven. Cool them on the baking sheet for handling.

SERVES 5

Prep Time: 40 minutes   **Cooking Time:** 15 minutes

Nutritional Facts: Calories 320, Total Fat 20g, Carbohydrates 6g, Protein27g

Ingredients

Pinch of crushed red pepper

½ teaspoon honey

½ teaspoon fresh lemon juice

1 teaspoon fresh cilantro

¼ cup Paleo yogurt substitute

1/8 teaspoon ground sumac

1 tablespoon extra virgin olive oil

¼ teaspoon saffron threads

¾ pounds grass fed ground lamb

¾ pounds minced turkey

1 lightly whisked egg

2 small ground garlic cloves

¼ teaspoon paprika

½ teaspoon minced black pepper

½ teaspoon crushed turmeric

¾ teaspoon sea salt

5 tablespoons Coconut Flour Bread Crumbs (refer to the recipe).

½ cup onion, grated

Directions

Place the grated onion over a sieve to take out the liquid and discard it. Start the grill on a medium high flame. Mix the onion, crumbs, salt, turmeric, black pepper, paprika, garlic cloves, eggs, minced turkey meat and lamb in a huge bowl. Shape the portions into rectangles and align a couple of pieces together on a skewer. Heat saffron for half a minute and crush it. Grill the kebobs and brush evenly with oil mixture and sumac. Serve with a blended sauce of Paleo yogurt substitute and the remaining ingredients.

SERVES 8

Prep Time: 50 minutes   **Cooking Time:** 15 minutes

Nutritional Facts: Calories 330, Total Fat 23 g, Carbohydrates 6 g, Protein 23 g

Ingredients

2 tablespoon olive oil

½ teaspoon saffron threads

½ teaspoon paprika

1 teaspoon ground turmeric

1 teaspoon freshly crushed black pepper

4 teaspoons sea salt

½ cup Coconut Flour Bread Crumb (refer to recipe)

2 lightly whisked eggs

2 chopped garlic cloves

1 pound ground sirloin (grass fed)

1 pound minced lamb (grass fed)

4 onions, grated

Directions

Place a sieve over a large bowl and fill it with grated onions to strain out the liquid that needs to be discarded. Set the grill on a medium high flame. Next mix the onions, bread crumbs, salt, turmeric, pepper, paprika, garlic, eggs, turkey and lamb in a sizeable bowl. Divide the meat into 20 portions and insert the skewers through them. Heat a small skillet over medium heat.

In a small pan heat the saffron threads for half a minute and crush this in a bowl. Mix it with olive oil. Grill the kebobs for 7 minutes. Brush the saffron mixture over these, sprinkle some sumac and use the rest of the ingredients to blend up a sauce. Once cooked, serve hot, with the sauce as the dip.

Ash-e-Reshteh (Special Persian Noodle Soup)

SERVES 3

Prep Time: 30 minutes   **Cooking Time:** 15 minutes

Nutritional Facts: Calories 360, Total Fat 19 g, Carbohydrates 37 g, Protein 12 g

Ingredients

1/8 cup fresh egg

1 tablespoon mint

8 sliced garlic cloves

2 cups zucchini noodles (thinly sliced into long curls)

½ bunch of chives

½ cup freshly chopped parsley

3 cups spinach

Black pepper to taste

Sea salt to taste

¾ tablespoons ground turmeric

¼ cup chopped cauliflower florets

1 sliced onion

¼ cup olive oil

Directions

In a sizeable bowl mix the salt, pepper, spices, breadcrumbs, parsley, garlic, onion and turkey. Take out portions and shape them into ovals. Refrigerate these for at least half an hour. For grilling, set the grill on high heat and insert the skewers into the meat and grill for around 13 minutes until the meat loses its pink color.

SERVES 3

Prep Time: 5 minutes + overnight and 3 days for marinating **Cooking Time:** 0 minute

Nutritional Facts: Calories 40, Total Fat 0 g, Carbohydrates 6 g, Protein 2 g

Ingredients

A healthy pinch of minced ginger

1 ¼ teaspoon sea salt

1 crushed garlic clove

½ cup celery slices

½ cup carrots

½ cup cauliflower

Directions

Put vegetables in water to soak overnight. The next day take a jar and mix ginger, garlic and salt in it. Add the vegetables and then finally add in the vinegar. Seal the jar and place in a refrigerator to marinate for 3 days at least.

SERVES 8

Prep Time: 3 minutes   **Cooking Time:** 1 hour 30 minutes

Nutritional Facts: Calories 340, Total Fat 16 g, Carbohydrates 46 g, Protein 5 g

Ingredients

¼ cup chopped walnuts

¼ cup walnuts

1 orange slice

1 lemon slice

1 small cinnamon stick

¼ cup honey

Syrup sauce (recipe below)

2 tablespoon olive oil

1 phyllo package, gluten free

¾ teaspoons crushed cardamom

1 cup chopped walnuts

Directions

First mix the cardamom, honey and walnuts. Grease a baking dish. Place a phyllo sheet on the work station, lightly rubbed with olive oil. Next align two tablespoons of the nut mixture lengthways on each phyllo. Fold the food strip with phyllo so that it looks like a single strip. Preheat oven on 350 degrees and bake for 35 to 40 minutes.

Now for the syrup: save the nuts and mix all the rest of the ingredients. Boil them and then when the mixture starts bubbling; reduce the heat to a simmer. Let it simmer for approximately half an hour. Let the food cool for 10 minutes and then pour it through a sieve. When the pastries come out of the oven, cover them with this strained liquid and let it soak in for an hour after which you may sprinkle pistachios and walnuts on top.

SERVES 17

Prep Time: 10 minutes   **Cooking Time:** 12 minutes

Nutritional Facts: Calories 130, Total Fat 7 g, Carbohydrates 16 g, Protein 1 g

Ingredients

¼ Oz nutmeg

¼ Oz cinnamon

¼ teaspoon sea salt

1/2 cup ground flax

½ cup almond flour

1 ½ tablespoon vanilla

½ cup coconut oil

1 egg

1 cup organic honey

Directions

Combine the wet and dry ingredients separately first then incorporate the two mixtures together. Align scoops of the cookie batter on a baking tray. Preheat Oven to 350 degrees and bake the cookies for around 12 minutes.

Walnut-Pomegranate Chicken

SERVES 4

Prep Time: 0 minutes   **Cooking Time:** 40 minutes

Nutritional Facts: Calories 200, Total Fat 8 g, Carbohydrates 7 g, Protein 25 g

Ingredients

Dash of crushed cinnamon

Pinch of saffron threads

1 teaspoon organic honey

¼ Oz tomato paste

½ cup pomegranate juice

½ cup homemade chicken broth

1 ground garlic clove

¼ cup finely diced onion

¼ tea spoon freshly ground black pepper

¾ teaspoon sea salt

24 Oz boneless chicken

½ cup toasted walnuts

Directions

Start by pulsing walnuts in a food processor. Next, season the chicken with salt and pepper. Take a large pot and heat it over a medium high flame. Next, toss in only half of the meat cook for around 3 minutes on each side and follow with the second batch of chicken. Now take a separate pan and sauté garlic and onion in it. Then sprinkle pinches of salt and pepper and the ground walnuts. Save the cilantro and toss in the remaining ingredients. Beat the food until the ingredients are mixed smoothly. At this point boil the food and at boiling point lower the heat to a simmer. You need to treat this as a reduction sauce. Give it around 15 minutes. After this duration add chicken to the pan and put on the lid and simmer for an additional 10 minutes. When ready, sprinkle with Cilantro on top.

SERVES 10

Prep Time: 20 minutes   **Cooking Time:** 20 minutes

Nutritional Facts: Calories 190, Total Fat 10 g, Carbohydrates 25 g, Protein 2 g

Ingredients

¼ teaspoon cardamom

¼ teaspoon saffron

1/8 cup rose water

½ cup natural honey

3 eggs

½ cup coconut flour

¼ teaspoon sea salt

2 Oz ghee

½ cup water

Directions

Boil salt, ghee and water in a sizeable non stick saucepan. Add the flour and continue stirring. Next, cut the flame to medium and keep on cooking, you will know when to stop when a dough ball forms and detaches from the bowl. Cool the victual for 10 minutes. Now replace the dough to a mixer and toss in the eggs, folding them in the dough one by one. Next, fill a pastry bag with this dough and line parchment paper on a cookie sheet. Squirt out the dough into the shape you prefer and bake the puffs for 18 to 20 minutes in a 400 degrees preheated oven. When the puffs are cooked and done cut them in half and fill the hollow cavity with honey.

Lamb Stew

SERVES 3

Prep Time: 15 minutes   **Cooking Time:** 7 hours

Nutritional Facts: Calories 398, Total Fat 20.7 g, Carbohydrates 6.6 g, Protein 44.2 g

Ingredients

¼ cup Paleo yogurt substitute

¼ cup water

1 carrot chunks

1 onion

2 tablespoon coconut oil

1 pound of boneless lamb shoulder (cut into cubic pieces)

½ a can of tomatoes

¼ teaspoon cinnamon

¼ teaspoon sea salt

1 teaspoon paprika

1 small dried chili

1 tablespoon coriander seeds

¼ tablespoon cloves

½ tablespoon green cardamom

1 red chili

½ tea spoon crushed black pepper

½ teaspoon turmeric

2 ground garlic cloves

1 ½ inch of ginger

Directions

Take a crock pot and stir together the ginger and garlic. Toss in the turmeric, pepper and Paleo yogurt substitute. Toss in the meat and coat it entirely with the rest of the ingredients in the bowl. Toast the cloves, cinnamon, coriander and cardamom. Blend onions with the chilies and the dried chilies then add the toasted spices to the blended onions along with the paprika in a small pan lined with coconut oil, and mix. Now pour this over the meat in the crockpot along with water, carrots, salt and tomatoes. Cook on a low flame for seven hours. Mix in the Paleo yogurt substitute once it is ready.

SERVES 4

Prep Time: 1 minute   **Cooking Time:** 0 minute

Nutritional Facts: Calories 150, Total Fat 0 g, Carbohydrates 49 g, Protein 2 g

Ingredients

Crushed ice as required

¾ cups organic honey

3 cups water

6 lemons

Directions

Juice half the lemons and thinly slice the remaining lemons. Put a sizeable saucepan over low flame and combine honey, water and lemon juice in it for 5 minutes. Next, drop the warm solution over the melon slices and cover with a cling film after which you need to refrigerate this for 4 hours. Stir through the water and serve with ice.

SERVES 28

Prep Time: 1 hour 10 minutes   **Cooking Time:** 25 minutes

Nutritional Facts: Calories 60, Total Fat 0 g, Carbohydrates 7 g, Protein 1 g

Ingredients

1 Oz crushed pistachio chunks (for garnishing)

¼ Oz rosewater

1 ½ teaspoon crushed cardamom

½ cup organic honey

1/3 cup extra virgin olive oil

1 ¾ cups coconut flour

Directions

Combine the flour, cardamom and honey. Eventually add oil to this, thoroughly mix and follow with rose water. Now pour the mixture into a pan and cover with cling film before refrigerating for 1 hour. When the dough is hard enough, take the pan out and cut up the dough with the cookie cutter of your choice. Next, put the cookies on a baking sheet and sprinkle with pistachio chunks. Bake for around 20 minutes in a preheated oven at 300 degrees.

Persian Maahi Kebabs

SERVES 8

Prep Time: 10 minutes   **Cooking Time:** 50 minutes

Nutritional Facts: Calories 420, Total Fat 29 g, Carbohydrates 8 g, Protein 32 g

Ingredients

2 lime

½ teaspoon pomegranate powder

1 teaspoon saffron

100 g mint (fresh)

2 Oz parsley (fresh for garnish)

100 g coriander

1 cup olive oil

1 cup lime juice (fresh)

8 large skinned fish fillets

Sea salt to taste

Black pepper to taste

Directions

Start by taking a sizeable bowl, mix in mint, parsley, coriander, salt, pepper, saffron, pomegranate powder, olive oil and lime juice. Take an oven proof dish and align the fish on it. Cover it with the sauce and put a sheet of aluminum foil on top of it. Bake this for around 45 minutes in an oven preheated at 180ºC. When cooked take it out of the oven and serve with lime slices and fresh chopped parsley.

Poached Eggs in Tomato Sauce

SERVES 8

Prep Time: 10 minutes   **Cooking Time:** 20 minutes

Nutritional Facts: Calories 150, Total Fat 0.2 g, Carbohydrates 37.6 g, Protein 0.3 g

Ingredients

2 tablespoon chopped chives

8 eggs

Sea salt and black pepper to taste

8 chopped tomatoes

2 garlic cloves

½ of an onion

¾ tablespoon olive oil

Directions

On a medium high flame, oil the skillet and stir fry the garlic and onions for 1 minute. Then reduce the flame to medium and keep on cooking for another 3 to 4 minutes. Toss in the tomatoes and simmer the food for 10 minutes. Without putting on the lid cook the food for another 10 minutes and sprinkle salt and pepper on top. Now once this sauce is nice and a bit thick. Scoop out 4 rounded portions (with the back of a spoon) in two batches and pour the insides of an egg in each of the dents. Cook till the eggs are done and serve with the sauce.

SERVES 8

Prep Time: 15 minutes   **Cooking Time:** 12 minutes

Nutritional Facts: Calories 467.1, Total Fat 37.1 g, Carbohydrates 3.9 g, Protein 27.6 g

Ingredients

½ teaspoon cinnamon

1 teaspoon pepper

1 teaspoon sea salt

2 eggs

½ of an onion, finely chopped

½ pound ground lamb (grass fed)

Directions

Start by taking wooden skewers and soaking them for around 20 minutes in warm water. Meanwhile, put the meat in a large bowl and toss in cinnamon, pepper, salt, egg and onion on top. Whisk the victuals thoroughly with a spoon until the meat's color gets lighter. Now take in a handful of mixture and fix it around the skewer in an elongated shape. If your meat is too wet to stick to the skewer just fold them in foil and grill them like that.

Grill the meat until it is entirely cooked and serve with lemon wedges.

Persian Carrot Salad

SERVES 12

Prep Time: 15 minutes   **Cooking Time:** 0 minutes

Nutritional Facts: Calories 170.2, Total Fat 10.7 g, Carbohydrates 17.8 g, Protein 3.3 g

Ingredients

1 teaspoon organic honey

1 teaspoon crushed cinnamon

2 teaspoon crushed cumin

2 Oz fresh lemon juice

2 Oz olive oil

120 g almonds

400 g apples, peeled and grated

1000 g grated carrots

Directions

Combine all the ingredients. Place in refrigerator at least an hour before serving.

SERVES 10

Prep Time: 20 minutes   **Cooking Time:** 40 minutes

Nutritional Facts: Calories 1176.3, Total Fat 93.5 g, Carbohydrates 23.9 g, Protein 64.7 g

Ingredients

5 tablespoons organic honey

6 cups pomegranate juice

4 cups homemade chicken stock

4 cups finely chopped walnuts

4 onions, sliced

6 pounds chicken

½ cup olive oil

½ cup lime juice

Sea salt to taste

Crushed black pepper to taste

Directions

Squirt the lime juice on meat and let it marinate for a couple of hours. Next, over a medium flame, heat an ounce. of oil. Now toss in the meat and make sure you brown it on all sides. Now toss in the onions and pour the remaining oil too; cook until the onions turn translucent. Mix in the walnut chunks and cook for another30 seconds. At this point, toss in the stock and the already browned meat. Bring the victuals to a boil, lower the flame and place a lid over it. It needs to simmer for around 20 to 25 minutes. Finally, mix in salt, pepper, organic honey and pomegranate juice. Simmer for an additional 20 minutes. Serve and enjoy!

SERVES 3

Prep Time: 10 minutes   **Cooking Time:** 0 minute

Nutritional Facts: Calories 89.2, Total Fat 0.4 g, Carbohydrates 20.4 g, Protein 1.9 g

Ingredients

1/2 Oz organic honey

8 Oz Paleo yogurt substitute

¾ cups red seedless grapes

Directions

Start by dividing the grapes into 3 portions evenly. Now do the same with the Paleo yogurt substitute. Layer 1/3 of the substitute on each portion and repeat the process with honey. Chill for a few hours before serving.

Khoresh Fesenjan

SERVES 12

Prep Time: 15 minutes   **Cooking Time:** 2 hours 30 minutes

Nutritional Facts: Calories 785, Total Fat 39 g, Carbohydrates 95.4 g, Protein 24.4 g

Ingredients

4 tablespoons organic honey

1 teaspoon cardamom

8 cups fresh pomegranate juice

2 teaspoon sea salt

1 pound walnuts

2 onions, finely sliced

3 pounds cut up chicken legs

4 tablespoons olive oil

Directions

Start by taking a large skillet and heating olive oil in it over a medium flame. Next, place the meat and onions in the skillet and cook the victuals for around 18 to 20 minutes. Now mix in the cardamom, pomegranate juice, sea salt and walnuts. Boil the entire mixture and reduce the flame to low. Put on the lid and let it simmer for 1 ½ hours. Do not forget to keep stirring the food. At this point stir in the organic honey and cook for another half an hour.

SERVES 3

Prep Time: 5 minutes   **Cooking Time:** 0 minutes

Nutritional Facts: Calories 442.5, Total Fat 12.7 g, Carbohydrates 84.2 g, Protein 8.1 g

Ingredients

½ cup almonds

½ cup fresh orange juice

½ cup figs, dried

1 cup pitted and chopped dates

1 banana, sliced

1 apple cored and peeled

1 orange, peeled and seedless

Directions

Start by choosing your salad serving bowl. Mix the orange juice and fruit gently, then sprinkle with almonds. Now cover the bowl, place it in the refrigerator, chill it for an hour, serve and enjoy.

SERVES 2

Prep Time: 20 minutes   **Cooking Time:** 15 minutes

Nutritional Facts: Calories 297, Total Fat 13.5 g, Carbohydrates 3.4 g, Protein 38.4 g

Ingredients

½ tablespoon sea salt

½ of an onion

1 pound beef tenderloin (grass fed)

1/8 cup fresh lime juice

Pinch of crushed black pepper

Directions

Start by chopping the meat into 1 ½ inch cubic pieces. Next add this to a mixing bowl with lime juice, black pepper, onion and sea salt. Mix thoroughly; make sure you cover the food before you place in the refrigerator overnight. Next, preheat the grill on very high heat and align the meat on the skewers. Now oil the grate and align the skewers with kebobs on the grill and cook for around 4 minutes on each side.

Yazdi Cakes

SERVES 12

Prep Time: 20 minutes   **Cooking Time:** 30 minutes

Nutritional Facts: Calories 215, Total Fat 14 g, Carbohydrates 19.9 g, Protein 3.4 g

Ingredients

¾ tablespoons pistachios. chopped

¼ cup blanched almonds, slivered

½ tablespoon rose water

¾ teaspoon crushed cardamom

½ cup Paleo yogurt substitute

¾ cups almond butter

2/3 cups organic honey

2 eggs

½ teaspoon baking powder

1 cup coconut flour

Directions

Start by mixing the baking powder and flour in a dry bowl and set aside. Next grease the indents of the muffin pan. Next take a heat proof bowl and mix the organic honey and eggs and put it on top of a pan filled with hot simmering water. At this point start whisking the mixture until it is white and pale. Give it at least 7 minutes. Now cut off the stove flame and keep on whisking the mixture for another 10 minutes. Stir in the rose water, cardamom, Paleo yogurt substitute and almond butter and mix thoroughly with your hands, eventually mix in the almonds too and fill them into the muffin molds. Top each muffin batter with pistachio chunks. Bake for half an hour in a 350 degrees oven. Take out, serve, and enjoy.

Ginger Sekanjabin

SERVES 2

Prep Time: 10 minutes   **Cooking Time:** 5 minutes

Nutritional Facts: Calories 601, Total Fat 0.6 g, Carbohydrates 150.4 g, Protein 1.1 g

Ingredients

¼ cup freshly ground ginger

¾ cups water

2 cups organic honey

Directions

Start by taking a sizeable saucepan and boil together the honey and water over a high flame for around 3 minutes. Then take the pan off the stove and mix in the ginger. Next let the mixture cool down a bit and sieve out the crushed ginger.

When using this syrup. Follow the ratio of 1 part syrup with 4 parts water.

SERVES 3

Prep Time: 2 minutes   **Cooking Time:** 10 minutes

Nutritional Facts: Calories 223, Total Fat 9.9 g, Carbohydrates 28. 3 g, Protein 6.2 g

Ingredients

1/8 cup organic honey

1/8 cup slivered blanched almonds

Rosewater as required

¼ cup almond chunks

3 cardamom seeds

1/3 cup arrowroot powder

Directions

Start by first dissolving the arrow root powder into ½ cup of chilled milk. Next, boil the remaining milk with almonds and cardamom. Now add the starch solution and continuously stir it with a whisking tool. At this point pour in the rose water and sugar to taste. Let the mixture boil for around 4 more minutes on a medium flame. Next take out the cardamom seeds and lay the rest of the victual on a serving dish. Finally sprinkle slivered almonds on top and serve hot or cold, any way you enjoy.

Iskender Kebabs

SERVES 8

Prep Time: 15 minutes   **Cooking Time:** 15 minutes

Nutritional Facts: Calories 667, Total Fat 36.2 g, Carbohydrates 48.6 g, Protein 37.3 g

Ingredients

½ cup freshly chopped parsley

½ cup Paleo yogurt substitute

1 cup ghee

Sea salt and pepper to taste

Crushed cumin as required or to taste

21.5 Oz tomato puree

2 ground garlic cloves

4 medium onions chopped

8 boneless chicken breast halves, skinless

1 Oz olive oil

8 coconut flour bread rounds

Directions

Start by lightly toasting the pita bread in the oven and then cut it into bite sized pieces. Next, take a skillet and heat the oil on a medium flame and toss in the garlic, onion and chicken. Eventually mix in the tomato puree and sprinkle it all with pepper, salt and cumin. Keep on cooking for an additional 10 minutes.

Now use a serving dish and at the bottom, layer it with paleo bread pieces. Sprinkle a bit of ghee on top and then layer it with the chicken. Use parsley and Paleo yogurt substitute as a final garnish.

SERVES 4

Prep Time: 20 minutes   **Cooking Time:** 35 minutes

Nutritional Facts: Calories 503, Total Fat 33.5 g, Carbohydrates 30.5 g, Protein 25.6 g

Ingredients

2 bunches fresh asparagus, sliced into an inch pieces

2 ground garlic cloves

2 cups water

12 Oz tomato puree

2 tablespoon turmeric, crushed

1 teaspoon crushed black pepper

1 teaspoon sea salt

1 pound lamb stew meat, diced

2 chopped onions

3 Oz olive oil

Directions

Take a saucepan and pour in the oil over a medium high flame. Next mix in the onions and cook for a minute or two. Remember to keep on stirring this mixture. Next add the turmeric, pepper, salt and lamb and cook the lamb until it loses the pink color on the outside. This will take around 3 to 4 minutes. Now mix in the tomato puree, garlic and water and let the food simmer, eventually cut the heat to medium low and cover the pan. Simmer for around 20 to 25 minutes.

Check to see whether the lamb is tender. If it is, chuck in the asparagus and keep on cooking for an additional 4 minutes.

SERVES 8

Prep Time: 5 minutes   **Cooking Time:** 20 minutes

Nutritional Facts: Calories 24.6, Total Fat 0.0 g, Carbohydrates 6.3 g, Protein 0.0 g

Ingredients

4 tablespoons organic honey

1 cup rose water

1 teaspoon crushed saffron threads

4 bruised green cardamom pods

8 cups water

Directions

Start by taking a kettle and put in the sugar, water, rose water and spices. Remember to stir this solution to ensure that the organic honey is entirely dissolved. First take the heat up until the solution boils then immediately lower the flame and let the mixture simmer for around 14 minutes. Serve after picking out the cardamom pods.

Khoresht-e-Hulu (Peach Stew)

SERVES 8

Prep Time: 5 minutes   **Cooking Time:** 1 hour

Nutritional Facts: Calories 551.7, Total Fat 27.8g, Carbohydrates 44.3g, Protein 32.5g

Ingredients

½ teaspoon saffron

6 peaches

1 cup organic honey

1 cup lime juice

1 teaspoon cinnamon

½ teaspoon cumin

1 teaspoon crushed cardamom

2 tablespoons rose water

½ teaspoon paprika

¼ teaspoon turmeric

1 ½ pound chicken breasts

2 Oz olive oil

2 large onions cut into rings

Directions

Trim the skin and fat from the meat and cut it into bite sized chunks. Take a non stick pan and heat it until it is lightly browned. Next, toss in the onions and oil. Now cook on a medium flame only until the onion goes translucent. Next, toss in salt and pepper, cinnamon, cumin, cardamom and rose water.

Now separately combine the saffron, sugar and lime juice and mix this mixture into the chicken. Cover the pot with a lid and let the food simmer for an additional 30 minutes. Next, cut the peaches into small wedges and mix them into the chicken meal. Cook for another 20 minutes.

SERVES 32

Prep Time: 30 minutes   **Cooking Time:** 0 minute

Nutritional Facts: Calories 34.9, Total Fat 0.6 g, Carbohydrates 7.3 g, Protein 0.3 g

Ingredients

¾ teaspoon vanilla

¼ cup tiny walnut chunks

1 cup organic honey

1/3 cup purred apricots, cooked first

1 Oz gelatin

Directions

Combine ¼ cup apricot puree and gelatin first and leave it for around 8 minutes. Put the rest of the puree in a saucepan and toss in the organic honey and boil the victual. Into this same bowl mix in the gelatin combination and simmer over a low flame for around 14 minutes. Remember to keep on stirring while it cooks. Stir in the walnuts and vanilla and lay it down on a pan to settle over night. Next morning, cut the meal into squares and toss them around in a bag of powdered organic honey.

Rose Petal Salad

SERVES 10

Prep Time: 35 minutes   **Cooking Time:** 0 minutes

Nutritional Facts: Calories 169.8, Total Fat 8.7 g, Carbohydrates 18.3 g, Protein 6.8 g

Ingredients

Freshly dried rose petal

Freshly crushed black pepper

4 ground garlic cloves, ground with sea salt

1 Oz freshly chopped fresh mint

4 tablespoons fresh dill

12 cup chopped walnuts

½ cup chopped green onion

6 cups Paleo yogurt substitute

2 cucumbers, peeled, seeded, halved (lengthways) and chopped in ¼ inch pieces

2/3 cup raisins

Directions

For half an hour soak the raisins in water. After draining them use a sizeable bowl and mix garlic, mint, dill, walnuts, green onions, paleo yogurt substitute, cucumber and raisins. Sprinkle salt and pepper on top of the mixture and place in the refrigerator for an hour. Before serving, garnish the meal with rose petal, mint, walnut and green onions.

SERVES 30

Prep Time: 10 minutes   **Cooking Time:** 15 minutes

Nutritional Facts: Calories 76.7, Total Fat 3.2 g, Carbohydrates 11.4 g, Protein 0.8 g

Ingredients

¾ raisins

1/16 teaspoon sea salt

¼ teaspoon crumbled saffron

½ teaspoon vanilla extract

2 large eggs

1 cup almond flour

¾ cup organic honey

½ cup ghee

Directions

Start by taking a mixer and combining ghee and organic honey until the mixture becomes fluffy. This will only take a couple of minutes. Whisk in the eggs. Next, blend in the sea salt, saffron and vanilla. After this, set your mixture to low speed and mix in flour. Next, mix in the raisins thoroughly.

Preheat oven to 350 degrees. Now, scoop the dough by a teaspoon and roll into petite balls. Line a baking sheet with parchment paper and align the balls on this. Bake these for around 10 to 11 minutes.

Recipes of Certain Ingredients to Refer to For the 50 Paleo Recipes

Paleo Coconut Flour Bread

SERVES 3

Prep Time: 5 minutes   **Cooking Time:** 45 minutes

Nutritional Facts: Calories 299, Total Fat 22.6 g, Carbohydrates 17.2 g, Protein 6.5 g

Ingredients

½ cup coconut flour

¼ teaspoon salt

1 tablespoon honey

3 whisked eggs

¼ cup coconut oil

1/8 cup coconut milk

Directions

Mix all ingredients together in a small dry bowl; pour in a baking tray lined with parchment paper and bake for 40 to 45 minutes in a 350 degree preheated oven.

SERVES 3

Prep Time: 5 minutes   **Cooking Time:** 45 minutes

Nutritional Facts: Calories 299, Total Fat 22.6 g, Carbohydrates 17.2 g, Protein 6.5 g

Ingredients

Paleo Coconut Flour Bread

Directions

If the bread is not dry enough to crumble into small pieces place it in the oven and bake it for around 10 minutes so that it is dry enough. Now tear the bread into small pieces and place these victuals in the processor and blend until you are left with the crumbs.

SERVES 3

Prep Time: 0 minutes   **Cooking Time:** 10 minutes

Nutritional Facts: Calories 228, Total Fat 23.1 g, Carbohydrates 5.3 g, Protein 2.2 g

Note: nutritional value with 1 cup cauliflower and 1 Oz Butter

Ingredients

Cauliflower florets (as required)

Grass fed butter (as required)

Directions

Take a food processor and blend the florets for a few seconds. Next transfer the chopped florets to a platter and combine it with the grass fed butter.

The Paleo Yogurt Substitute

Serves 3

Prep Time: 5 minutes   **Cooking Time:** 13 minutes

Nutritional Facts: Calories 184, Total Fat 19.1 g, Carbohydrates 4.4 g, Protein 1.8 g

Ingredients

1 cup Coconut Milk

1 tablespoon Gras fed gelatin

Squeeze of lime juice (fresh)

Directions

Mix half of the coconut milk with gelatin and set aside. Next, take a sauce pan and combine the rest of the coconut milk with lime juice and once it starts heating reduce the flame to low and pour in the gelatin paste. Refrigerate this.

When you are ready to use this, put the set yogurt alternative in a food processor and puree until it is smooth again.

Final Word: The Persian Aroma

Persian culinary differs accordingly with the occasion. With their preserved history come the age old authentic recipes of Persia in modern day Iran. It must be acknowledged that the ingredients chosen in each meal was chosen carefully to balance the nutrients and ultimately, the health benefits. There is little wonder in why they meals incorporate so much of the vegetables and herbs.

Every recipe in this book has been created for all those Paleo lovers who want variety in their life. These recipes will not only tantalize your taste buds, but also give you a taste of true Persian cuisine, no matter in which part of the world you reside. Test your culinary prowess, give these recipes a try and lose yourself in this Persian blend of delectable and mouthwatering meals.

So what are you still waiting for? Embark on this journey of fragrant spices, healthy ingredients, and amazingly divine dishes. Follow the recipes provided in the book and experience the true flavor of Persian food, in Paleo style!